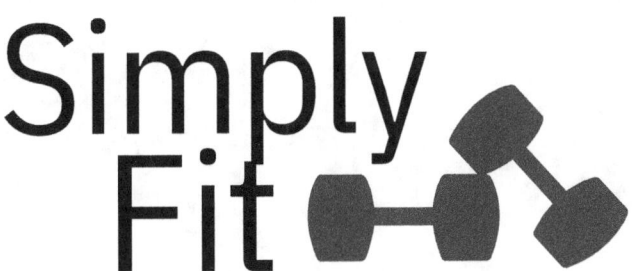

# Simply Fit

*If you would've started your workout when you first thought of it, you would be fit by now.*

Janae Neuville

Janae Neuville

ISBN:1517108543
ISBN-13:978-1517108540

Simply Fit

Simply Fit

# <u>Warming up</u>

Warming up keeps your body injury free. A light five minute warm up before beginning any workout or sports activity can help avoid injuries.

Warm up Example: Stand with your arms out by your side and make small circles five forward five backwards and repeat

Even something simple like jumping rope or doing calisthenics:

- Increases muscle temperature for improved stretch.
- Increases blood flow to working muscles
- Proper workouts will improve performance.

# Stretching

The best way to stretch is slow movement. If you bounce while stretching, it can cause an injury because your muscles will tighten, not relax. Hold your stretch for about Ten to Twenty seconds. Repeat 2 or 3 times. Try to extend the stretch each time .There should never be pain while you stretch. Don't force the stretch. Your body needs time to loosen each muscle group.

 Here are some Stretching Examples:

Lower leg stretch

Standing groin stretch

Butterfly stretch

Side lunge stretch

Front lunge stretch

Trunk twist stretch

Flamingo stretch

Calf stretch

Ear to shoulder stretch

# Fitness WorkOuts

Repeat all Routines at least twice for beginners Let reps depend on fitness level.

## Full Body Blast Workout

25 Lunges

30 Squats

25 Side lunges

25 Pistol squats

35 Calf raises

30 Crunches

45 Wall sits

20 Jumping jacks

50 Dumbbell split jump

25 Leg lifts

40 Sumo squats

35 Bicycle crunches

35 Leg raises

30 Russian twists

25 Squats

# Butt Workout

25 Shoulder bridges

10 Jump squats

24 Squats

20 Jump lunges

20 Clam

30 Side lunges

25 Shoulder bridges

40 Deadlifts

20 Plie  squats

10 High heel shapers

25 One leg bridge

20 Single leg bridges

# Butt Blast Workout

25 Jump lunges

30 Inner thigh leg lifts

25 Shoulder bridges

20 Donkey kicks

20 Fire hydrant

35 Hip lifts

20 Donkey kicks

25 Table top pull back

25 Shoulder bridges

## Quick Workout

Step up with leg lift 1x20
Reverse lunge with front kick 2x20
Lateral leg lift 3x20

# Cardio workouts

## 2 reps, 30 second rest between

10 Climbers

25 Speed skaters

10 Shoulder taps

15 Tricep dips

10 Burpees

25 Planks

25 High knees

20 Jumping jacks

25 Crunches

30 Jump squats

10 Butt kicks

25 High knees

15 Side to side jumps

15 Sprinter sit ups

# <u>Intense workout</u>

## 2 reps, 30 second rest between

45 Jumping jacks

45 Squats

40 Mountain climbers

25 V sits

25 Push-ups with rotation

25 Planks up & Down

30 Flutter kicks

35 Cross crunches

2 Minute wall sit

# Core Workouts

- Trunk flexion

crunches, quick torch toe touch, full sit up,

weighted crunch, medicine ball toss twist crunch.

- Hip flexion

leg raise circle, leg thrust, leg raise, straight leg raises.

- Rotary Torso

half bicycle, twisting sit-up, leg press down (Leg press

down, lie on the floor on your back with legs straight

up.Your partner will stand facing you with their feet on

each side of your head. Your arms are bent and your

hands are holding your partner's ankles for stability. Your

partner pushes both of your legs straight down toward the

floor. Resist and stop the downward movement as quickly

as possible without feet touching the floor, then with your

straight legs quickly return to the starting position, your

partner will repeat the push down.

# Strength Training

Always Adjust the equipment and weight to fit your body and individual needs for every exercise.

## **Bar Squat**

Place the bar on the rack just under your shoulders so that you have to squat slightly to place the bar on the back of your shoulders. Stand with both feet and hips under the bar. Straighten your legs to lift the bar off the rack. Get into position; stand slightly wider than the hips and toes pointed out. Keep your eyes, head and chest up maintaining a tight back throughout the lift

## **Leg press**

Lie in the leg press with your back flat and your butt touching the pad slowly push the weight up keep your butt on the pad and your back flat at all times

## **Standing calf raise**

Stand with your feet on the calf machine platform, heels down, calves stretched and body straight. The pads are on your shoulders, raise on your toes as high as possible and hold for count return to the starting position.

# <u>Workout Routines</u>

- Alternate dumbbell curl

- Barbell curl

- Wrist curl reverse

- Curl concentration

- Curl dumbbell

- Curl tricep workout

- Tricep pushdown

- Overhead tricep extension

- One arm dumbbell extension

- Dumbbell tricep extension

- Overhead barbell extension

- Seated barbell extension

- Abdominal crunch

# Three Major Gluteus Maximus Muscles

| Medius | Jumping Jacks |
|--------|---------------|
| Maximus | Lunges |
| Minimus | Squats |

## Gluteal Muscles

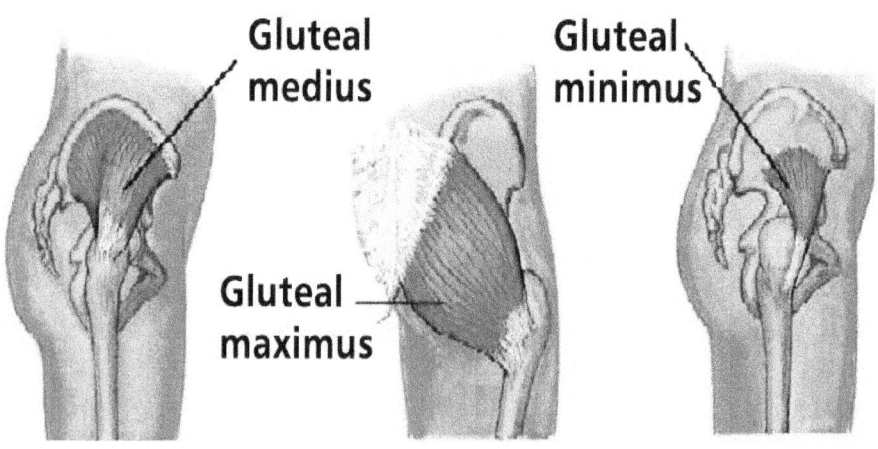

# Things To Know
## Facts and More.

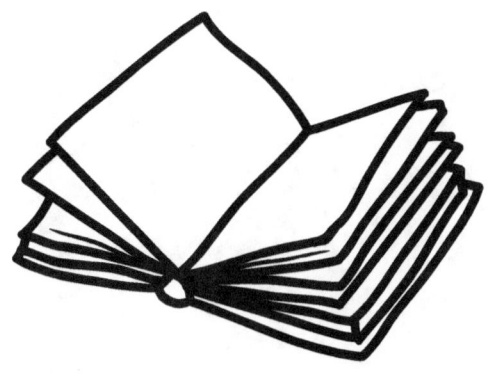

# Acidic Vs Alkaline

Before starting something new you need to figure out which direction to go. So why not educate yourself?
Healthy tissue in the body is alkaline and acidic food is cancerous tissue in the body is Acidic. Knowing the difference will help you transition over to a healthier lifestyle.

| Acidic Foods | Alkaline Food |
| --- | --- |
| * Red Meat , Poultry & Seafood | * Fruits & Vegetables |
| * Dairy Products | * Millet |
| * Grains,Flour & Breads | * Nuts & Seeds |
| * Artificial Sweetener & Sugars | * Dark, Leafy Greens |
| * Condiments | * Herbs & Spices |
| * Processed & Fast Foods | * Beans & Legumes |

# Alkaline

-

### High Content

Stevia, Celery, Kelp, Kale, Parsley, Collard greens, Mustard greens, Green Bell Pepper, Spinach, Avocado, Artichoke, Asparagus, Cayenne pepper, Broccoli, Sprouts, Wheat Grass, Veggies, Chard Greens, Herbal Tea, Watermelon, Chlorella, Straw Grass, Alfalfa Grass, Blended Greens Drink.

### Moderate Content

Okra, Cabbage, Radish, Onion, Garlic, Tomato, Ginger, Basil, Lemon & Lime, Oats, Quinoa, Sauerkraut, Lentils, Wild rice, Almonds, Chia seeds, Lettuce & Arugula, Chives, Butter & Soy Beans, Haricot Beans, Green tea, Figs, Pears, Sorrel, Cumin seeds, Raw Almond Butter, Baking Soda, Cilantro, Oregano, Cantaloupe.

### Low Content

Cauliflower, Zucchini, Red Potatoes, Lentils, Olive Oil, Coconut Oil, Flax oil, Carrots, AlmondButter, Milk, Squash, Grapefruit, MInt, Hemp seeds, Fennel seeds, Ginger Tea, Chestnuts, Kamut, Cinnamon, Apple Cider, Ginseng, Sprouted Bread & Wraps.

# Acidic

## High Acidic content

Alcoholic beverages, Carbonated Drinks (Soda) , Coffee, Energy Drinks, Sweetened fruit juice, Prunes, Chocolate, Veal, Turkey, Mussels, Lobster, Shrimp, Beef, Tuna , Sardines, Shellfish, Cod, Preserves, BlackBerries, Black Tea, Vinegar, Pork, Soy Sauce,Bacon,Lard.

## Moderate Acidic content

WholeGrains, CranBerries, Apples, Papaya, Dates, Pomegranate, White and Brown Sugar, Corn tortillas, Sourdough, White Bread, Duck, Chicken, Buffalo, Salmon, Cheese, Butter Margarine , Sparkling Water, Bananas, Mandarin, Raspberry, Pineapples, Brown Rice, Cheese, Barley, Ketchup, Mayo, Mustard, Cereal, Canned fruits.

## Low Acidic content

Sunflower oil, Chickpeas, Liver, Rice milk, Whey Soy Protein Shake,Yellow Plums, Couscous, Rye Bread, Basmati Rice, Cashews, Walnuts, Macadamia Nuts, Sweet Potatoes, Pecans, HazelNuts, Ice Cream, Pinto beans, Pumpkin seeds, Processed Honey, Molasses, Oats, Pasteurised fruit juice.

# <u>You eat better , You feel better</u>

## Super foods that benefit the Human Body

**Eyes**

Corn, Eggs, Carrots, Oranges, Kale, Spinach, Green Beans.

**Heart**

Tomatoes, Potatoes, Prune Juice, Citrus fruits, Oatmeal, Grits, Salmon.

**Bowls**

 Prunes, Yogurt, Blackberries, Garbanzo beans, Whole Grain.

**Bones**

Oranges, Celery, Yogurt, Milk, Cheese, Spinach, Wheaties.

**Brain**

Walnuts, Blueberries, Salmon, Tuna, Sardines, Walnuts, Whole Grain products, Brown rice, Bread, Tortilla.

**Muscle**

Cottage cheese, Red meat, Fish, Eggs, Bananas, Cashews, Almonds, Protein shakes.

# Food Facts

**Eggs** a good source of protein and vitamin B

**Spinach** will help keep your hair shiny

**Whole grains** have zinc iron and vitamin B

**Apricots** are a good source of vitamin A

**Vegetarians** turn to flax seeds for a Omega-3

**Potatoes** are a rich source of carbohydrates

**Chicken breast** is said to be the healthiest nonfat part

**Beans** are a good protein substitute for vegetarians

**Bananas** are rich in carbs and a great workout fuel

**Pineapples** keep your gums healthy

**Cherries** calm the nervous system

**Omega 3** contain anti-inflammatory properties

**Grapefruits** are the leading fat burner along with

having a great source of vitamin C.

# <u>Benefits of Spinach & Broccoli</u>

- Helps the brain and nervous system function

- Strengthens bones

- Promotes healthy glowing skin

- Strengthens the immune system

- Helps improve vision

- Lowers high blood pressure

- High levels of antioxidants

- Anti-inflammatory

- Helps prevent diabetes

- Boosts immune system

- Helps with diabetes

- Fights heart disease

- Promote healthy bones

- Regulate blood pressure

- Regulate hormones

# Clean Eating Grocery Guide

## Fruits and veggies

Apples, Bananas, Clementine, Cherries,

Grapes, Strawberries, Peaches, Avocados,

Blueberries, Raspberries, Romaine lettuce, Celery,

Carrots, Spinach, Sweet potatoes, Cucumbers,

Corn, Bell peppers, Kale, Tomatoes,

Broccoli, Zucchini, Squash, Artichokes.

## Dairy

Unsweetened almond milk, Horizon organic Brand,

Greek yogurt, Cottage cheese, Gelato,Cage free eggs,

Organic eggs, Low fat shredded cheese.

## Grains

Brown rice, Whole grain bread, Whole wheat pasta,

Whole wheat wraps, Whole grain English muffins.

## Meat

Chicken breast, Turkey bacon, Turkey breast, Tuna.

# Carbs , Fats and Protein

*All three groups provide energy for the muscles.
*Protein helps build tissue
*Carbs are stored in the Muscle and Liver
*Fat is the Primary source of Energy

## PROTEIN

Salmon, Turkey, Chicken, Eggs, Greek yogurt, Tuna, White fish, Whey protein powder, Cottage cheese.

## Vegetarian Alternatives

Peanuts, Dried Beans, Green Beans, Peas, Edamame seeds, Sun-Flower seeds.

## Carbohydrates

Whole grain bread, Whole grain tortilla, Berries, Apples, Quina ,Beans, Oats, Brown rice, Sweet potatoes.

## Fats

Almonds, Coconut oil, Avocado, Flax seeds, Chia seeds, Pecans, Olive oil, Almond butter, Peanut butter ,Salmon.

# Carbs Carry Both Sugar And Starch

## Bad Carb Examples:

White flower, White bread, Muffins, Pretzels, Rice, Pastry Pancakes, Potato chips, Fries, Hot dogs.

## Bad Sugar Examples:

Juice candy, Sugar, Soda, Jelly, Honey.

## Bad Starch Examples:

Bread, Muffin, Crackers, Pasta, Rice, Potatoes.

**This is an example list. There are more items in each category for you to continue to educate yourself to be on a great path towards avoiding all unnecessary and unwanted carbohydrates.**

# Food Low In Sodium

## Food Known for the low levels of sodium

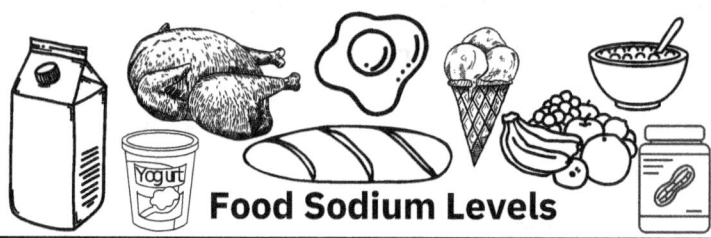

**Food Sodium Levels**

| | |
|---|---|
| 2 tbsp of Peanut Butter | 0.050mg |
| 1 Egg | 0.060mg |
| 1 oz of Chicken | 0.020mg |
| 8 oz of Milk Or Yogurt | 0.125mg |
| ½ Cup of Ice Cream | 0.050mg |
| ½ Cup of Fruit | 0.015mg |
| ½ Cup Of Vegetables | 0.010mg |
| 1 Slice of Bread | 0.150mg |
| 1 oz Wheaties Cereal | 0.250 mg |

# Simply Fit

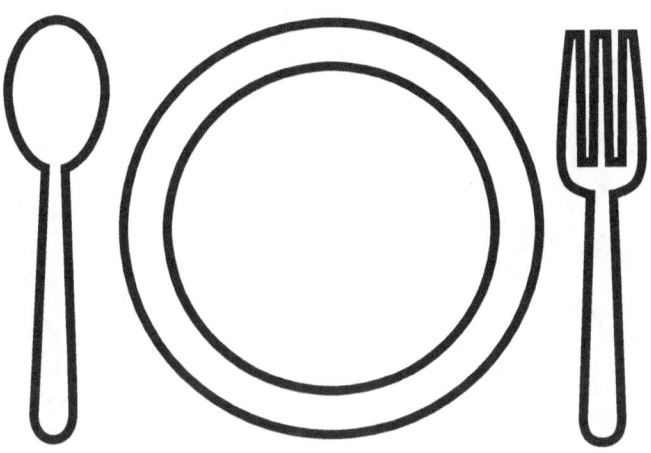

# Healthy Recipes

## Janae Neuville

# <u>Sauteed Green Beans</u>

## **Ingredients**:

1.Fresh green beans

2.Coconut oil (refined) or Olive oil,

3.Garlic powder, Onion powder and Salt & Pepper.

## **Prep**:

Cut off the ends, boil until soft, once green beans are done drain water.

## **Cook**:

Add olive oil or butter, whichever you prefer, into the pan. Put boiled green beans in the skillet with the stove on low to medium. Season to taste.

# Cajun Baked Chicken
## Stuffed With Spinach & Cheese

## Ingredients:

1.1 pound boneless skinless chicken breast

2.Feta cheese

3.Spinach

4.Avocado oil

5. Cajun spice, Sea salt & Pepper

## Prep:

Cut chicken breast diagonally. Place the cheese and spinach inside where you just made the cut. Add a tablespoon of oil on top of the chicken breast then season to taste. Wrap in aluminum foil.

**Cook Temperature:** 350 degrees **Bake Time:** 30 to 45 minutes

# Baked Lemon Chicken
## With Collard Greens And Brown Rice

## Ingredients:

1. Chicken thighs or breast

2. Lemons sliced for Garnish & Lemon juice

3. Garlic and Onion powder

4. Sea Salt & Pepper

5. Collard or Mustard Greens

6. Brown rice

**Prep**: Place chicken in a shallow dish. Season to taste with salt & pepper.Put the lemon juice on the chicken, add slices of lemon on top as a garnish.

**Cook Temperature:** 350 degrees  **Bake Time:** 25 to 45 minutes

# Baked Salmon and Asparagus

## Ingredients:

1. Fresh skinless salmon filets

2. Asparagus (Slim)

3. Avocado oil

4. Minced garlic two cloves, Parsley & Basil

5. Blackened pepper, Paprika and Sea salt

## Prep:

Place fresh salmon in the middle of aluminum foil. Sprinkle a small portion of oil then season to taste with garlic salt, fresh ground pepper, one lemon thinly sliced with a piece of parsley. Place asparagus on top of the complete salmon and fold in aluminum Foil. Place in oven

**Cook Temperature:** 350 Degrees **Bake Time:** 45 minutes

# Mozzarella Grilled Cheese
## <u>With Spinach and Garlic</u>

## Ingredients:

1. Italian bread or Texas toast bread

2. Fresh mozzarella cheese

3. Avocado oil

4. Garlic clove

5. Baby spinach and Baby arugula leaves

## PREP:

Set the skillet to medium heat. Add oil evenly to coat pan then saute minced garlic, spinach and arugula together until wilted. Remove and add sautéed food with the mozzarella to your bread or wrap of choice.

**Cook:** Heat pan on medium heat and add sandwiches cook to your desire on each side.

# Customize your own trail Mix

## Nuts:

Cashews, Pecans, Almonds, Peanuts, Walnuts or Pistachios.

## Dried Fruit:

Blackberries, Banana chips, Cranberries, Cherries, Apricots, Peaches, Raisins and Apples.

## Seeds:Sunflower, Pumpkin or Flax.

## Sweets:

M&Ms, Chocolate chunks, Marshmallows or Peanut Butter brittle.

## Grains:

Granola, Pretzels, Popcorn, Mini Wheaties, Cheerios ,Life cereal or Yogurt covered pretzels.

# A Healthy Sweet Tooth

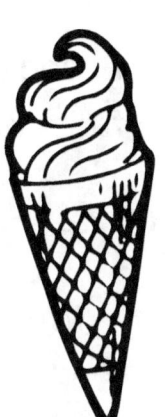

Freeze your favorite yogurt put into a jumbo waffle cone, garnish with almonds and strawberries.

Cut two bananas into small pieces, put in the freezer after three hours, remove and put into a blender, blend well and serve.

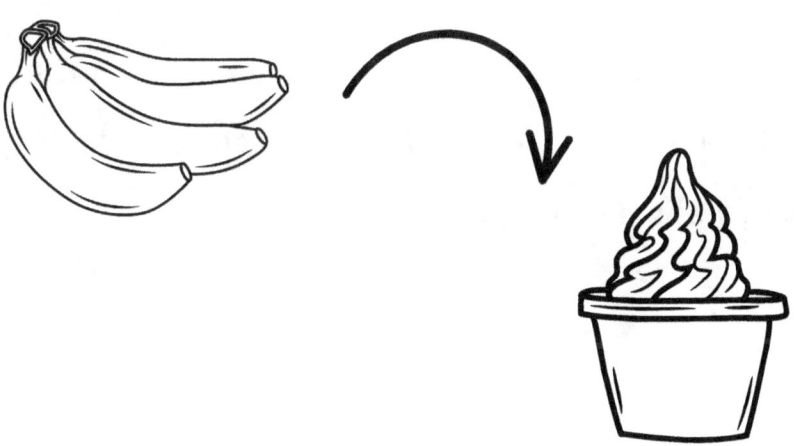

# Fit Facts

Based on a moderately active lifestyle, how many fruits & veggies do you need?

| Gender/Age Group | Daily Average Intake |
|---|---|
| Women | 4-5 Cups |
| Men | 5-6 Cup |
| Teen | 4-5 Cups |
| Kid | 3-4 Cups |
| Toddler | 2 Cups |
| Senior | 1-2 Cups |

## Weight Loss Tip

To lose a pound of fat each week you will need to burn 500 or more calories a day than you consume, this may require some calorie counting and tracking.

# What Do You Know About Water?

- Water regulates your body temperature

- Removes waste

- Composes 75% of your brain

- Makes up 83% of your blood

- Composes 22% of your joints

- Makes up 75% of your muscles

- Helps the body absorb nutrients

- Protects and cushions your vital organs

- Converts food into energy

- Moistens oxygen for breathing

- Water helps carry nutrients and oxygen to cells.

# Detox Drinks

## Directions:

When preparing detox waters, let the end result sit in the fridge for 3 hours. Leave overnight for best results.
Good for 2 days.

## Detox Benefits

*Drop up to 10 lbs with detox water drinks.

*Helps flush out harmful toxins in the blood.

*Mint aids in digestion

*Cucumbers contain anti-inflammatory properties

*Ginger is a natural pain reliever and aids digestion

*Lemon helps combat harmful toxins

*Helps weight loss

*Has antioxidants

*Toxin cleanser

**Toxin:** A poisonous substance, especially a protein, that is produced by living cells or organisms. They are capable of causing diseases when introduced into the body tissues but are often also capable of inducing neutralizing antibodies or antitoxins.

# <u>Detox Water Recipes</u>

4 Cups of water
1/2 Cup cherries
1/2 Lemon, sliced
1/2 Lime, sliced
1/2 Kiwi, sliced

4 Cups of water
1/2 Cucumber, sliced
1 Cup strawberries
1 Cup blueberries

4 Cups of water
1 Mango, sliced
1 Cup strawberries, sliced
1 Cup oranges, sliced

4 Cups of water
1 Kiwi, sliced
1 Cup blueberries
1/4 Cup of pineapples

4 Cups water
1 Red apple, sliced
1 Peach, sliced
1 Kiwi, sliced

4 Cups water
1 Plum, sliced
1/2 Lime, sliced
1 Cup blackberries

4 Cups water
1 Mango, sliced

Janae Neuville

# Detox Bath Recipe

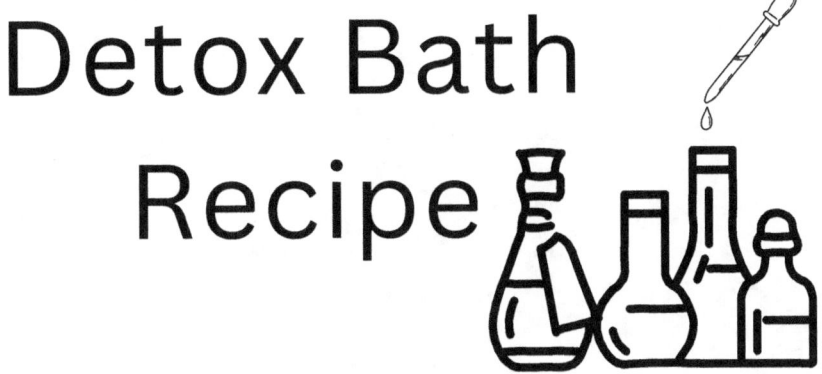

# Natural Spa Treatment

Once a week, for 20 minutes, soak in a hot bath that contains 1 to 1.5 cups of Epsom salt or Sea salt. Add 10 to 15 drops of lavender essential oil and ½ cup of baking soda. These three things combined together draws out toxins,lowers stress related hormones and balances pH levels.

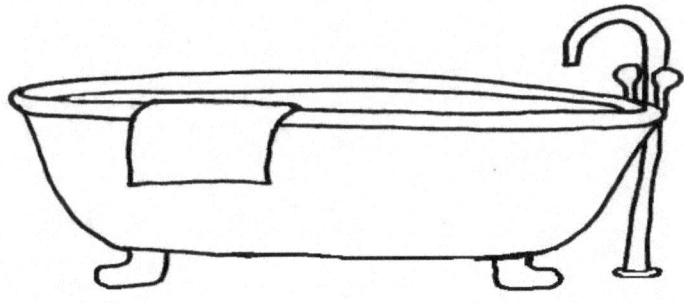